Unisex
Toilet Retraining

Unisex
Toilet Retraining

Urinating Sitting Down
Produces Clean Toilets.
Urinating Standing Up
Creates Smelly Filthy Unsanitary Toilets

Anthony Seymour Browne

Mr. Anthony Seymour Browne
P.O. Box 365
New Rochelle, New York, 10802
U. S. A

Browne, Anthony Seymour
        Unisex Toilet Retraining

ISBN 978-1492934356

Cover & Book Design by Pub-My-Book.com

Author photo credit: PROphoto Studio, Sheraton Mall, Barbados

Disclaimer and Reader Agreement

Reader Agreement for Accessing This Book

Dedication

In1968, I had the insight to toilet train myself to urinate sitting down and enjoy a clean bathroom at home.

Early in 2013, some extraordinary events converge. First, I discovered Taiwan and Sweden have proposals encouraging men to sit down and urinate. Second, I learned why urinating standing up messes up bathrooms are because of the urethra and tip of the penis. Third in 2013 the tools for self-publishing is abundant. Fourth, my Divine Theocratic Education adequately qualifies me to research, write and publish for the benefit of others.

Proverbs 4:18 states. "The path of the righteous ones is like the bright light that is getting lighter and lighter until the day is firmly established." Men sitting down and urinating and producing clean toilets is an idea that is getting brighter and brighter.

Such timing and circumstances are much greater and bigger than me, or any other human. That is why I give all credit and thanks for my unique circumstances and this book, to my all knowing Creator Jehovah, God.

Table of Contents

What is Unisex Toilet Retraining?

Unisex Toilet Retraining is a concept the author pioneered. Unisex means appropriate to both sexes, and not distinguishing between male and female. Toilet Retraining means males changing from the traditional model, urinating standing up to urinating sitting down using the same position as females. Then, both genders will be using the unisex home toilet as designed and not as a gender-specific toilet since it is not. We will now explain why this toilet retraining is necessary.

Why is Retraining Necessary?

To appreciate why toilet retraining is necessary, we have to face the facts that public toilets or bathrooms for men are filthy, with puddles of urine on the floor and horrible urine odors. What's more, the condition is an international problem and the cause is men standing up to urinate.

In an effort to clean up their country's public toilets: Sweden and Taiwan have proposals encouraging men to sit down to urinate. Could such proposals soon lead to unisex toilets? This question may not be too farfetched.

Unisex Toilets and Restrooms

In many countries, unisex bathrooms are fulfilling an urgent requirement on privacy for all. Worldwide, there is an increasing aging population. Also, there is an increase in various debilitating illnesses and deteriorating physical conditions. That is why it is commonplace to see someone caring for the restroom needs of another person of the opposite sex. Who could be a marriage mate, life-partner, parent, child, caregiver or a friend?

Those situations require Unisex Toilet Facilities, with privacy. Gender-specific facilities cannot adequately care for those unique needs. Without men accepting retraining, those Unisex restrooms will become filthy like the current Men's Only Restrooms. Clearly toilet retraining is necessary and becomes evident by the current proposals encouraging men, to sit down, to urinate.

Proposals Encouraging Men to Sit Down and Urinate

Taiwan and Sweden have proposals encouraging men, to sit down and urinate in public toilets.

Taiwan: "Men should sit down to urinate in the toilet instead of standing up because it helps maintain a cleaner environment." Says, Stephen Shen the Taiwan's Minister Environmental Protection Administration (EPA) Department.- Aug 28, 2012.

Sweden: Left Party wants men to pee sitting down. Published 11 June 2012 07: 10 CET "Men, who work for the Sörmland County Council in central Sweden should sit down rather than stand up when urinating in office toilets, according to a motion, put forward by the local Left Party Chapter."

A look back at history and current events reveal why the proposals are not a laughing matter.

Proposals to Sit Down And Urinate Are Not a Laughing Matter

The proposals for men to sit down to urinate are not a laughing matter. Especially when we look at the following four relevant points:

1. The history of Sweden as a pioneer regarding the health issue

2. The history of United States Department of Agriculture, health objective

3. The comprehensive research study by the Taiwan Environmental Protection Administration

4. Urinating, a frequent occurrence, and the enormous volumes of urine.

Sweden's Leading Role, On Health Issues

First, history records Sweden's leading role, on health issues. For example, the first food pyramid was published in Sweden in 1974. The most widely known food pyramid introduced by the United States Department of Agriculture in the year 1992. Was updated in 2005, and then replaced in 2011. Over 25 other countries and organizations have also published food pyramids. Source: Food guide pyramid, From Wikipedia, the free encyclopedia.

Please note Sweden took the lead role in the world way back in 1974 to publish a food pyramid with better health as an objective. Then later in *1992* the United States Department of Agriculture (USDA) developed its first food pyramid.

The United States Department of Agriculture, Health Objective

The United States Department of Agriculture has a health objective, to prevent obesity, chronic diseases and dental diseases. This food pyramid had revisions in 2005 and a replacement in 2011. This latest food pyramid is now, the most widely known food pyramid in the world.

The second key point is history also shows in the interest of improving human health, and well-being the United States Department of Agriculture (USDA) revised established dietary and nutritional practices.

What is undeniable, today, over 25 other countries and other organizations, also have food pyramids. On this current health issue will other countries also follow Sweden.

An Objective And Comprehensive Research Study

The third point is this, the Taiwan proposal results from an objective and a comprehensive research study by their **Environmental Protection Administration (EPA)**. This review of 100,000 **inspections of public toilets is a large** population and the conclusions are significant. Who then can ignore such a detailed report?

Urinating Frequent Occurrence And Significant Volumes

The fourth point is urinating frequent occurrence and significant volumes of urine. On the matter of frequency, most adults urinate about once every two to four hours when awake and for a total of about six to eight times in a 24-hour period.

Furthermore, the volume of urine is also astounding. The U.S. National Institute of Diabetes and Digestive and Kidney Diseases reports, adults typically produce about one and half quarts, about 1.4 liters, of urine daily, with the bulk of production occurring in the daytime. However, this amount can range significantly, from just under a quart to half a gallon, 800 milliliters to two liters, daily. That translates into enormous quantities of urine in developed countries and astronomic amounts worldwide.

Enormous Quantities In Developed Countries And Astronomic Amounts Worldwide

Let us do the maths at the low end of the statistic, one and half quarts, about 1.4 liters a day. Multiply one and half quarts or 1.4 liters times the number of adult males in each developed country who stand up to urinate. Then it is reasonable to understand and contemplate, the enormous quantities of urine disposal in an unsanitary way in those countries and the astronomical daily amounts worldwide.

Add to that fact this key point. Urinating demands attention and refuses postponement even for a few hours and certainly no indefinite postponements. Those factors provide the large picture and places urine disposal in the proper perspective.

It is obvious, anything that occurs daily and with such frequency and flows in such enormous quantities and demands immediate attention and refuses postponement; deserves the best practices. More importantly, it is a serious matter that demands attention.

Whereas, it is common practice for blogs, forums, chat rooms and some websites to discuss the proposals for men to sit down and urinate as just a joke. However, as the foregoing shows the proposals for men to sit down to urinate are not a laughing matter.

The next topics look at the jokes on the Internet relating to urinating sitting down. "Real men do not sit down" and "bashing penis and dipping the penis in water."

Unisex Toilet Retraining

Why is it Real Men Sit Down to Urinate?

Why is it real men sit down to urinate goes contrary to a common objection, "Real men don't sit down." The proponents of this latter statement, often say: sitting down is effeminate. Also sitting down to urinate makes a male look like a sissy. It is not manly. Does not show masculinity, that he has a penis and he is a man.

The Author Relates

"At my niece Andrea's home, her ten year old son Russell came into the bathroom. He sees me sitting down on the toilet and asks, Uncle Tony what are you doing? My reply, I am peeing. Russell's immediate response, **"Uncle Tony, you don't have a penis?"**

The main point. At age 10 years, his idea is a male should stand up and urinate because he has a penis."

9

Factually, how does one show he is a man? Is it only by the simple act of standing up to urinate whether at home or in a gender-specific toilet?

Here is a beneficial side bar, which shows one act, does not define gender. The Genesis account teaches that man was out of the woman. Did that make Adam a sissy? Here, is what happens afterward: "For although the first woman came out of the man, all men have been born from women ever since, and both men and women come from God." -- 1 Corinthians 11:12 The Living Bible.

This is the main reason why the real men sit down to urinate they want to keep the bathroom at home clean.

Keep The Bathroom Clean

Real men sit down to urinate at home because they want to keep the bathroom clean and presentable at all times. Whether they live alone, or share the home with other female relatives: wife, mother, sister or friend. Please remember women like to keep immaculate clean homes. Sitting down will save several million women around the world from cleaning up toilet urine odors.

It is true women often find their toilet or bathroom to be the dirtiest and their biggest source of embarrassment. How do we know?

When we visit a home and ask the female of the house, to use her bathroom. She usually replies, give me a minute. Then off, she goes to perform a smell test and a quick look at the bathroom. This is especially the case when a boy(s) or a male(s) share the home.

Why the hasty inspection to make a quick check? This allows her time to make the toilet tidy for the visitor's use and prevent embarrassment. Some men share the same sensitivity and also value a clean toilet. A toilet without urine odor is the reason why real men sit down to urinate.

The second objection to sitting down to urinate is the fear of bashing the penis while shaking and also dipping the penis into the water.

The author's personal experiences.

Sometimes when peeing my urine was not going into the toilet bowl. When I see the urine start going off track, I would stop urinating and then start again. Thinking my urine stream would somehow self-correct.

At other times, I would stop urinating and pinch the end of my penis and start urinating again. Reasoning that my urine flow would become laser-like and go straight into the bowl. Those strategies and techniques to control my urine stream were not successful.

On occasions, I still continue to spew urine on the bathroom floor. However, a day in 1968 I wet my feet. That is when I said, enough and started to sit down to urinate.

Up to this date, I still sit down to urinate because I want to get my urine into the toilet bowl and so have a clean bathroom at home.

Unisex Toilet Retraining

Fear of Bashing Penis and Dipping Penis Into Water

Some men fear bashing the penis while shaking. Also dipping the penis into the water of the toilet bowl. As a result, they are reluctant to accept sitting down to urinate. So let us visit both issues.

First, as discussed later under the topic "Milking The Urethra," a male should not be shaking his penis after he finishes urination. Instead, milking the penis is more efficient than shaking the penis, because milking accomplishes the objective, which is to remove extra urine from the penis. Therefore, toilet retraining makes bashing the penis a moot issue.

Second, concern of dipping the penis into the water of the bowl. Sitting down to urinate is the same as sitting down to defecate. The penis is usually in the same position for both elimination processes. So it is reasonable to suggest doing the same thing when sitting down to urinate as he does when having a bowel movement.

Furthermore, dipping the penis into the water with feces is a more serious issue that dipping into the water with urine. Since, fecal matter should never come into contact with other parts of the body. Please consider these two practical and easy solutions.

Two Practical Solutions

The first practical solution is to purchase a raised toilet seat. This provides more height and distance from the water in the toilet bowl. Plus it is better for tall persons and those with painful knees. The second practical solution is, when sitting down on the toilet hold the penis as formerly when standing up. Both suggestions will prevent dipping the penis into the water.

Consequently; the fear of shaking the penis and hitting the toilet bowl and dipping the penis into the water of the toilet are not compelling reasons to refuse to sit down after reviewing the following points.

Shaking the penis is a moot issue. Men navigate the water when sitting down for a bowel movement and can do the same thing when sitting down to urinate. They can also hold the penis as if standing up to urinate. The other alternative is to purchase a raised toilet seat.

Some men have one mind set, and want to maintain the tradition of urinating standing up.

The Tradition of Urinating Standing Up

Some men want to maintain, the tradition of urinating standing up. An article in the Japan Today News and Discussions, dated Friday March 15, 2013, by Philip Kendall on the topic, "Standing up to pee 'a matter of honor' for one man" illustrates the strong emotion for his tradition. In addition, it also shows how men insist on standing up although it leads to marital strife. Please Google the article and have an entertaining read.

There are many voices on the issue and also the pros and cons of urinating sitting down. One thing is certain the practice of standing up is from the tradition, of times past and teaching by a mother, grandmother, nurse, nanny or child-rearing expert(s), or by modeling Dad, uncle or older brother. The fact is the same teacher(s) also passed on the tradition of sitting down for a bowel movement.

Does, urinating at that time and in the sitting position, make him a lesser man or feel less masculine? Also, he does not have to stop sitting down and stand up to urinate, and then sit down again, does he? As we think about it, we discover when we sit down it is a normal comfortable experience. Thus, a desire to stand up to urinate is a head thing due simply to tradition.

Urinating Standing up is a Head Thing

Urinating standing up is a head thing. Why so? Every time the same objector sits down to ease his bowels he proves he can also sit down and urinate. Since, he also urinates at the same time. So a person needs to ask himself what are the benefits of him standing up? Then in the light of his answer, he may see his only obstacle to urinating sitting down is a head thing. Fair enough?

More importantly, tradition must be weighed on the scales of proper hygiene and the demands of a modern society. In this 21st century, standing up to urinate as a tradition does not promote up-to-date good hygiene, either at home or in a public toilet.

Practice Good Hygiene

How to practice good hygiene at home? Well, sitting down to urinate promotes good hygiene. Why would a reasonable person choose to stand up and urinate and in the process spray, spill and spot up his pants and immediate surroundings?

When there is the best option to sit down and get his urine safely into the toilet bowl: every time, everywhere, every place and at every age. Those terrific outcomes are only some of the many benefits of sitting down to urinate.

Many Benefits From Urinating Sitting Down

It is true there are many benefits from urinating sitting down. Men seldom give any thought to the subject and continues doing as taught during childhood without considering how it impacts his life and the life of others. In this modern age, there is a better way.

Sitting down to urinate is smart. Among other things, prevents spray and spill on the pants and urine on the floor, the toilet seat and the bathroom walls. Gets rid of smelly urine odors in toilets. Eliminates the need for disgusting and continuous cleanups. Guarantees getting urine into the toilet bowl every-time regardless of age. To appreciate how those benefits come about, we must compare a urinal and a home toilet bowl.

Compare Urinal and Home Toilet Bowl

Compare a urinal and a home toilet bowl on design and function. The design of a urinal is for males to standup to urinate in public places. On the other hand, the design of a home toilet is for bowel movement and not urination.

Why is that distinction beneficial? Urinals have a back-splash and a wall. Yet, the toilet floor and surrounding area get splatters, spills and sprays; when men stand up and urinate.

Could standing up to urinate at home, have a different conclusion than standing up at a urinal? Remember the home toilet design is for sitting down. So if, men stand up to urinate at home, where is the back-splash and the wall? The raised toilet seat: lid, hinges, and the rim become substitutes for the back-splash, and wall of the urinal and they get the urine that goes astray.

Granted in a home there is not the volume of urination as in a public place. Although that is so, even small amounts of urine such as tiny droplets, little squirts and delicate sprays, produce excellent growth medium for bacteria. Urine waste breaks down and infects every place urine lands, with smelly urine. This creates an unsanitary toilet and a hygienic disaster. What if, your partner dislikes the smell of urine and also hates to clean it up.

Partner Dislikes Smelly Urine Odor, Hates Cleaning Urine

What should a man do, if he realizes his partner dislikes smelly urine odor and hates cleaning it up? Also, she is sick and tired of continuously trying to get rid of urine odor in the bathroom? That is why women want men to sit down when peeing. We have to face the fact, many persons dislike cleaning urine. Doing so is unpleasant. A task that a wife and partner does not want to perform.

Imagine how much more detestable doing so becomes, when it is a continuous problem. For example, here's a quote from a wife: "I clean my bathroom regularly, but a day or so later, I can always smell urine. I clean in and around the toilet good, but the odor still comes back." **APA:** Urine Smell in My Bathroom | ThriftyFun. (n.d.). Retrieved from http://www.thriftyfun.com/default.ldml?tf_index=tf10792249&redirect=true&search_mode=1

Under those circumstances, it is only natural for this woman to vent her feelings. Since, she wants to have a bathroom without the smell of human urine. As seen in **France** and **Germany** and **Holland.** "The liberated woman of France and Germany and Holland has vowed to put their men - down on the toilet. They carry placards showing a huge red X scrawled across a man standing to urinate. The shout in France 'Drop your trousers and sit!' In Germany, 'Keep your drips to yourself' and Holland 'Not another filthy puddle on MY bathroom floor!' "

APA: To sit or not to sit - The Naked Scientists. (n.d.). Retrieved from http://www.thenakedscientists.com/HTML/articles/article/to-sit-or-not-to-sit/ For good reason, then, a male needs to ask himself, why is he still standing up to urinate? Especially if, he wants to end the most common complaint against him and stop the quarrels.

End, Common Complaint Against Husbands

Sitting down and urinating is the best way to end the most common complaint against husbands, which is, the mess they make while peeing. Sitting down is the only proven practical solution to aim urine into the toilet bowl without messing the floor, the toilet seat and the lid. So a wife cleaning up urine would not exist.

As a result, a wife has less work and more time for other matters, including her husband. In addition, here are some other benefits. It makes the wife happy. Eliminates quarrels on a painful issue and fosters a better relationship. She sees her husband respects her feelings, and the husband resolves the basis of the most complaints; thus, ending the constant quarrels.

According to a Dong-A Ilbo survey of 500 single people conducted Monday and Tuesday via Sunwoo, a marriage consulting company, 230 men (46 percent) said they will sit down to urinate for their wife while 85 (17 percent) were doing so. Sunwoo CEO Lee Woong-Jin said, "This is Men's voluntary choice in consideration of their wives at home."

Besides that, there is the remedy for three troublesome ongoing issues. First, eliminating a source of ongoing quarrels. Second, spraying urine on the toilet seat, bowl or the floor. Third, making someone continuously cleaning up urine odors.

Unisex Toilet Retraining

How to Get Rid of Cleaning Toilet Urine Odors at Home

Many women ask how to get rid of cleaning toilet urine odors at home. Most people think getting rid of recurring odors are an impossible task, but that is not the case.

To be successful follow these three simple steps:

- Identify the source of the urine odor.

- Isolate the main cause.

- Provide a practical solution rather than encourage the process.

Identify the Source and Main Cause

How to identify the source of the urine odors is easy. Who are the primary users of the bathroom? They are usually residents of the home, close family, relatives, friends, acquaintances and visitors.

What is the main cause of urine odors in the bathroom? Universally, it is males urinating standing up. Clearly we isolate the primary source of urine odors in the bathroom, correct? This is the very essence of how to get rid of cleaning toilet urine odors at home.

Please look carefully at the combination of the source and the main cause of the urine odors. What is essential to know, few aspects of life cause more pain or frustration or heartache or joy than dealing with this intimate group of people. Some housewives attempt to provide a practical solution by making requests on how people should use their bathroom. They apply stickers and posters and hang plaques in their bathroom.

Popular Bathroom Stickers

The lists of the popular bathroom stickers' decals come in different statements and applications. Some stickers are for applying to bathroom walls and the toilet bowl and the seat. Others are for the bathroom door entryway, and they read as follows.

- If you sprinkle while you tinkle, be a sweetie and wipe the seatie.

- Put me down bathroom seat decal.

- I aim to keep this bathroom clean.

- My aim is to keep the bathroom clean. Your aim would help.

- Our aim is to keep this bathroom clean - Gentlemen - Your aim will help, please stand closer -- it's shorter than you think!

- Boys, our aim is to keep the bathroom clean. Your aim will help.

Are these the best practical solutions for preventing cleaning toilet odors? Not at all, but rather poor ideas and for several reasons and how so? Because, they encourage males to urinate standing up: the primary reason of urine odors in private toilets and also public toilets worldwide. The Taiwan Government Environmental Protective Agency comprehensive research study of over 100,000 public toilets offers undeniable proof regarding public toilets.

The second reason why those popular bathroom stickers are not the best practical solutions is that they do not outright reject raising the toilet seat. Instead, they speak about the "aim and put me down and stand closer and when you sprinkle." Clearly these are encouraging peeing in the standing position and "be a sweetie and wipe the seatie" is also problematic. Wiping the seat with only a tissue leaves a film of urine and bacteria breaks down. This infects every place urine lands with smelly urine odor. (Click here to read more about **seat up issues** and see the long lists of negative outcomes when men raise the seat.)

Consequently, women desiring a clean bathroom are defeating their purpose with some popular bathroom stickers encouraging peeing standing up. The practical solution should get rid of cleaning toilet urine odors at home rather than producing the urine odors.

Only Practical Solution That Eliminates Odors

There is only one practical solution that eliminates odors and prevents cleaning toilet odors. It is a solution like the proposals of

Sweden and Taiwan governments: encouraging men to sit down to urinate in public toilets. That is why the author suggests this practical slogan. "Unisex Toilet Retraining Urinating Sitting Down Produces Clean Toilets. Urinating Standing Up Creates Smelly Filthy Unsanitary Toilets." This slogan identifies the problem and provides the solution and gets rid of urine odors instead of causing the odors.

Plus, this powerful message is a straight forward statement for a housewife who dislikes cleaning toilet urine odors should display. The buyer beware notice at the point of sale cash register informs shoppers on the company's refund policy. Similarly, the bathroom notice informs toilet users on the home owner's policy.

What New Bathroom Sticker Accomplishes

The new bathroom sticker expresses the different outcomes between sitting down and urinating standing up. Standing up creates smelly filthy unsanitary toilets and sitting down produces clean toilets. This unique notice accomplishes several things with that statement.

- How the owner wants to avoid cleaning urine odor.

- Educates what works at their home.

- Expresses the cause of filthy and clean toilets.

- States the personal values of the home.

- Allows people who use the bathroom to express their compliance with the wishes of the owner(s).

If a home displays such a notice in the bathroom and a male enters the bathroom, then suddenly his urine sounds like a waterfall. First thought that he is urinating standing up. The second is that he disrespects the house rules for a clean toilet.

Disrespect House Rules for Clean Toilet

Some people disrespect or disregard the house rules and owners in some unusual ways. Here is how some may feel about your home when they use the bathroom.

"I usually sit and pee at home and good friends' homes. Whenever I come to the place of someone I don't like or disrespect, I stand and pee because I don't give [an expletive] about the hygiene of their place."

APA: Peeing sitting down | Is It Normal? | http://isitnormal.com. (n.d.). Retrieved from http://isitnormal.com/story/peeing-sitting-down-920/

How will one know if those using their home have a similar disposition? Unless people using the bathroom have a physical challenge sitting down, you will know this when, after seeing the express wish, they continue urinating standing up. Such behavior shows direct disrespect and violates the rules of the home.

At this point let us discuss a crucial matter, and show how the design of the penis makes urinating sitting down the only perfect option. We will illustrate this fact, using a pilot of a ship.

Unisex Toilet Retraining

Pilot Directs Ship But Not His Urine

A male pilot directs a ship but cannot direct his urine, because of two factors. Both relate to design and function; on the ship it is the rudder on the penis it is the urethra.

Regarding the ship The Living Bible makes this point at James 3:4: "A tiny rudder makes a huge ship turn wherever the pilot wants it to go, even though the winds are strong."

What is the key fact? In this case, the design of the rudder in relation to the ship. So that the pilot, perhaps after only a few months training, masters the technique, steers and docks a large ship. He can successfully perform the task, even if he is at the helm of the ship for the exact first time.

Could the pilot stand up and direct his urine into the toilet bowl at home, with the same success rate he controls and docks his ship?

The answer is no. Although, he has more practice with his penis than with the ship his lifetime of practice does not help him.

Lifetime of Practice Does Not Help

Why, a lifetime of practice does not help the pilot with his aim? What contributes to his success with the ship is the design of the rudder and how it functions. Likewise, the pilot's inability to steer his urine in the direction he wants it to go, is also due to the design of his penis, and how it functions.

When the pilot sets the rudder for his ship to go straight, the ship would not go to the left or right. It would not. On the other hand, when this pilot aims his penis for his urine to go straight into the toilet bowl, the urine may go to the left or right and miss, no matter how hard he tries to direct or correct his urine flow.

Has such, been also your personal experience when urinating? This is an extremely crucial point for every male to understand. What causes him to miss the toilet bowl. Why he cannot direct and control his urine flow, is due to the design of the penis.

Design of The Penis

The design of the penis contributes to a male's inability to direct his urine. It is vital ALL men get this fundamental point and understand the reason. Dr. Levine of Men's Health Magazine says: under his topic: "You aim straight it pees left."

"Why does your urine stream sometimes takes a left turn into the bathtub? The problem is your meatus, or the tiny opening at the tip of your penis. Urine spirals out of your urethra like a bullet out of a gun," says Dr. Levine. "If there's dried mucus, ejaculate, or any other irregularity in the meatus, it can make the stream split or go off-center."

Therefore, a key reason why men cannot get their urine to go into the toilet bowl is because of the design of the penis. On the other hand, men with poor eyesight, half asleep or blind can sit down and do better. So here are some experiences.

Partially Blind, Half-asleep Or Blind

Men who are partially blind, half-asleep and blind benefits from sitting down to urinate. They sit down in complete darkness and get their urine into the toilet bowl. Better than a man with 20/20 vision urinating standing up in the full light of day.

The foregoing makes a powerful statement, why men should sit down to urinate, is that not true? Here, are some real-life experiences.

"I was a clerical worker and also driver for a company. Then it all happened. Cloudy eyes when I awake in the morning. Plus, the invoices did not seem as clear as formerly. When driving, I saw the vehicles coming towards me, but I could not clearly identify the license plates.

As a result, I went to an ophthalmologist who diagnosed Glaucoma. My eyesight gradually deteriorated. All my life I stood up to urinate, but as my sight faded sometimes I sat down and other times I stood up.

Then in 2004 while standing up and urinating, I realized that I was wetting my feet with urine. From that time, I decided to sit down to urinate because I did not want my wife cleaning up my urine from the toilet floor.

As of this date March, 2013, my vision is only two percent in the right eye and zero percent in the left eye. In this partially blind condition, I sit down to urinate. It is the only way I can use the

toilet to urinate, without messing up the toilet with urine." –
A. Alleyne, Barbados, West Indies.

Here is an experience of a man half-asleep...

"I pee sitting down especially when I go during the middle of the
night. No, aiming and worrying about peeing all over the floor while
still half asleep, it just makes sense." **APA**: Peeing sitting down |
Is It Normal? | http://isitnormal.com. (n.d.). Retrieved from
http://isitnormal.com/story/peeing-sitting-down-920/

In addition, some men experience issues directing and controlling
the urine flow.

How to Direct and Control Urine Flow

How to, direct and control urine flow become an issue in the following situations. The lack of force to urine flow makes directing the stream difficult. On other occasions, the urine squirts in a direction not intended. This sprinkles the floor, the toilet, seat and wets the pants with urine. Another problem to overcome is urine drainage and dripping. Worst of all is the common habit of shaking the penis to get rid of residual urine. All results, in stale urine odor, whether in the bathroom or on the trousers.

What is the solution? Retraining in urine elimination. Urinating sitting down prevents some of those issues. Here is how. First, sit down to urinate. Second, milk the urethra. Thus, he eliminates urine in the penis after he finishes urinating. This practice helps empty some urine that remains, usually the primary cause of pants wetting after urinating.

It is advisable that if dripping and drainage continues it could be due to some medical condition. Since that topic is beyond the scope of this book, men should visit an Urologist if the problem persists.

Now back to the extremely relevant topic, the vital retraining milking the urethra and sitting down.

Milking The Urethra

A vital aspect of toilet retraining is milking the urethra. "A press behind your scrotum, can help you avoid dotting your trousers, or you can use a technique called urethral milking. Simply run your finger along the underside of your penis to force out remaining liquid," says Dr Fishman. -- Words by *Men's Health*.

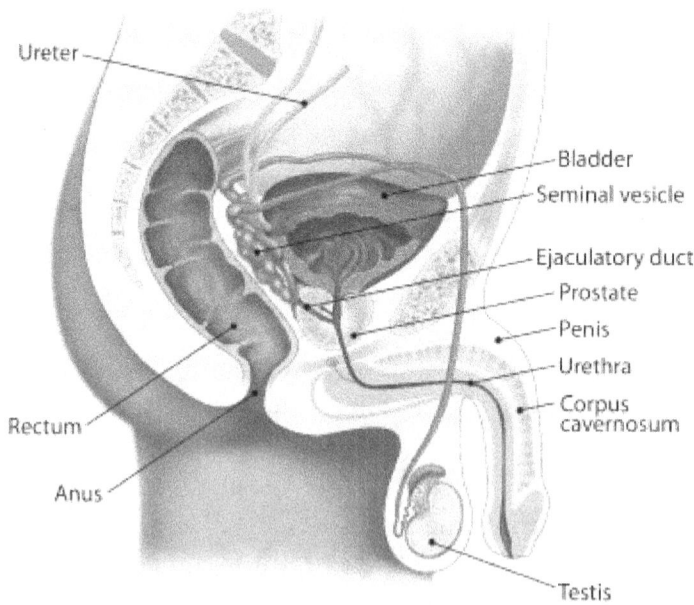

Please take a close look at the picture of the urethra. The shape and position reveal why it is highly unlikely shaking a penis will eliminate all the residual urine from the urethra. On the other hand, running the finger along the underside of the penis is more likely to force out remaining urine.

That is why it is also beneficial to sit down. Place toilet tissue at the tip of the penis and milk the penis. This catches the extra urine that otherwise would end up in the underwear or on the trousers and also eliminates the need to shake the penis. A practice that contributes to sprays, and urine odor in toilets. Another advantage to proper urine elimination is to avoid what traps urine in the penis.

What Traps Urine in The Penis

What traps urine in the penis? When a male stands up to urinate through his pants fly, the fly pushes up against the urethra and traps his urine. On the other hand, when he sits down to urinate and drops his pants he has unrestricted urine elimination. Please take another look at this book's cover. Notice the person who is sitting drops his pants. Whereas, the person who is standing is peeing through his pants fly.

Please think seriously about those two facts, because the dead last thing a male wants to do is to trap his urine. The design of the penis already presents a challenge emptying the urethra and trapping urine makes the penis embarrass a man.

The Penis Embarrasses a Man

The penis embarrasses a man. This little body member. Spots up the toilet with droplets when it drips. Scatters sprays on the floor when shaken which produces an excellent growth medium for bacteria. This sets the wheel of natural life of the organisms aflame, the breakdown of products stinks and provides a hygienic disaster.

This process creates a continuous defeat for a female trying to keep a urine odor-free toilet or bathroom. The primary reason is how urine flows from the bladder and through the urethra and into the tiny opening at the tip of the penis. That is what directs the urine flow, not the man with the penis in his hand.

That is the precise reason a male cannot standup to urinate and consistently get his urine stream under his control. The only way to save embarrassment from his penis is to stick with the basics of toilet retraining.

Stick With the Basics

It is necessary to stick with the basics of toilet retraining. This retraining is the process of learning the new skills. As already discussed, some basics include sitting down and urinating and milking his urethra. Other new skills are wiping the tip of his penis rather than shaking it trying to eliminate urine. Also, always sitting down to urinate, instead of standing up, all qualifies as retraining.

What is different about unisex toilet retraining for a male. The cost is zero, no extra time, effort or hard work. He is not changing anything he enjoys and doing anything he dislikes. Neither is he starting changes his body requires getting accustom to on a short-term or long-term basis. Toilet retraining is not like that at all, but rather a healthy lifestyle change.

A Healthy Lifestyle Change

It is true a healthy lifestyle change usually takes time, effort and discipline. The body must adapt to the new lifestyle. This is a common experience with losing weight, dieting, quitting smoking and stopping alcohol consumption.

Although, maintaining those lifestyle changes are difficult many persons succeed. However, this new healthy lifestyle change is uniquely different. Why is that statement true? The body eliminates urine in the sitting position when a male sits down to have a stool.

As a result, there is only one significant change. Instead of sitting down just for bowel movement, he also sits down to urinate. Occasionally a life-threatening health issue requires serious lifestyle changes to save a life and people accomplish those changes.

Granted, standing up at home to urinate is not life threatening. However, if a male asks his wife, mother, girlfriend, or a female in the home which she prefers him do at home stand up to urinate, or to sit down.

The happiness she shows at his consideration will surprise him. Imagine how much more so, if he follows through and starts immediately and continues unwaveringly? Because his body teaches him doing so, is easy.

What the Body Teaches

What is it the body teaches that makes it easy to accept urinating sitting down? The world's most renowned designs and inventions result from studying living things and how they work. The most advanced and efficient living thing is the human body. What does the body teach?

Here is a key lesson. Whether male or female, toddler or adult, the human body teaches the same lesson. The elimination process of excrement and urine usually accompany each other.

What is more, when having a bowel movement at home a man sits on the toilet and also urinates in the sitting position. In addition, the body teaches other undeniable and amusing lessons.

Undeniable Amusing Lessons

These undeniable and amusing lessons males experience on several occasions are lesson one: he feels he wants to have a bowel movement. So he sits down on the toilet seat, but instead of the bowel movement, he passes gas and urinates while still sitting down on the toilet.

He accomplishes relief, and his body provides a clear signal, and he has no more feeling for the bowel movement. The lesson he learns is he can sit down and urinate.

Lesson two, he feels he wants to urinate and stands up to do so. While standing, he has a sudden urge for a bowel movement. Does he insist he is standing up to urinate, and that is exactly what he will do and have the bowel movement afterward.

Absolutely not! He would not even dare attempt to urinate at that crucial time. Rather, he will speedily abandon the standing position and obey the urge for the bowel movement. Otherwise, he will mess himself. What is even more intriguing, after he sits down, he will have the bowel movement and also urinate.

So there it is! His body teaches and makes it easy for a male to accept sitting down to urinate. Different undeniable and amusing lessons, for sure. The benefits of toilet retraining are also evident with the effects of advancing age.

Effects of Advancing Age

The effects of advancing age attacks the body and leaves a trail of conditions that require men to sit down to urinate. The wise King Solomon writing under inspiration describes what happens to the human body. He writes, "For there will come a time when your limbs will tremble with age, and your strong legs will become weak, and your teeth will be few to do their work, and there will be blindness, too." Ecclesiastes 12:3 The Living Bible.

A fact of life and we see those same conditions on a daily basis. Perhaps in a male relative: a grandfather, father, uncle, brother or cousin. A dearly loved family member is at that same stage in his life.

His hands and his legs tremble, due to weakness and nervousness. The eyes, coupled with their mental faculties by which they see— are dim, if not totally dark. In that condition toilet retraining, sitting down to urinate, is better than standing up. It prevents him from messing up the bathroom floor.

What can we do to help? Tactfully go over the various points in this book on toilet retraining and highlight the several benefits of sitting down to urinate. Also assure him that his condition is not Parkinson's or Essential Tremors, and he is only experiencing the effects of advancing age.

Men Who Have Tremors

Men who have tremors benefits from toilet retraining. It is common for tremors to occur with sufferers of Parkinson's and Essential Tremor conditions.

Parkinson's disease is a common movement disorder with an estimated worldwide prevalence of 6.3 million people. Source: European Parkinson's Disease Association (EPDA).

"Essential tremor is 5-10 times more common than Parkinson's disease. An estimated 10 million Americans suffer with a neurological disorder called essential tremor." Source: Harvard School of Medicine, Family Health Guide.

What is the difference between those two conditions? Many people associate tremors with Parkinson's disease, but the two conditions differ in key ways: "Essential tremor of the hands usually occurs when you use your hands. Tremors from Parkinson's disease are most prominent when your hands are at your sides or resting in your lap." Source: Mayo Clinic Staff.

Here are some vital statistics.

"Approximately 1.5 million people in the U.S. who suffer from Parkinson's disease - approximately 1-2% of people are over the age of 60 years." Source: The American Parkinson's Disease Association.

"Essential tremor can occur at any age and is most common in people age 40 and older." Source: Mayo Clinic Staff.

Urinating standing up, and holding his penis would be difficult for a man with tremor of his hands. That is why learning to sit down through toilet retraining benefits men who have tremors as it helps with *hygiene and cleanliness.*

Hygiene, Cleanliness and Health

Taiwan history will show that hygiene and cleanliness and health are the main reasons for the country's proposal. Taiwan's environmental protection agency objective in proposing men to sit down and urinate. Is to promote good hygiene and cleanliness and better health and to ensure that men do not, step through puddles of pee.

Here, we have indisputable evidence from the Taiwan study. Standing up to urinate is unclean, unhygienic and unhealthy. With that in mind, what is the position at home?

What is the Position at Home?

What is the position at home is an appropriate pun. It could mean, where we stand on the issue. Or literally what is the posture at home standing-up or sitting down to urinate.

This is a predicament all men face, because if a man thinks he can stand up to urinate. Then shake his penis as he performs the ritual learned during potty training; without messing up the toilet. He is just fooling himself. Somewhere a sprinkle(s) will fall.

What is to be done with the common practice of urinating? Change to a method that prevents sprinkles and sprays and urinating sitting down is the best option. This also applies to one-toilet establishments.

One-Toilet Establishments Proper Toilet Etiquette

The major issues with one-toilet establishments are cleanliness and proper toilet etiquette. Since both genders use the same toilet or bathroom, it is a Unisex Toilet. These facilities are what we use on buses, trains, airplanes, bars and some hotels, restaurants, and small businesses and small offices.

In these toilets, the issue revolves around men and how they use the restroom. The core problem is mostly men standing up to urinate. Where, the toilet has deposits of urine, on the seat or floor.

In other instances, some men raise the seat to prevent spraying, but then forgets to lower the seat. In either case, the one-room toilet is not in the best condition for the next person, whether male or female.

How a Restaurant Responds

How a restaurant responds to the unsanitary conditions in their one-toilet establishment. In Vancouver, Canada a restaurant bans men from peeing standing up. If other one-toilet establishments will follow the same option, nobody knows for sure.

One thing is certain, men standing up to urinate presents issues and challenges to cleanliness and proper sanitation. Perhaps the concept of the golden rule, leaving the bathroom in the condition suitable for the next person, is a good idea to keep in mind.

Paying it forward in this respect changes the whole mindset and makes using one-toilet establishments a pleasant experience for both sexes. The best way to start is by unisex toilet retraining. Which means at home, and other unisex toilets such as one-toilet establishments using the unisex toilets in a unisex manner. Both genders urinating sitting down and correcting the main defect of standard boys' toilet training.

Standard Boys' Toilet Training Defects

Standard boys' toilet training defects start during potty training and continues throughout a man's life time. The chief defect is that method's BIG contributions to unsanitary toilets all over the world. It is often said, insanity is doing the same thing again and again and expecting different results.

That is why rational thinking people ask, why is it we still toilet train little boys to stand up and pee, why this training? What are the benefits of training boys to urinate standing up? There is overwhelming evidence, from all over the globe that urinating standing up produces unsanitary conditions.

It disturbs to discover the disgusting habit results after extensive, traumatic, extra training for both mother and little boy. Furthermore, when we take a close look at the training process it is contrary to fundamental logic.

For example, we first train a little boy to sit down on the potty to ease his bowels and to urinate. He masters that skill and he supposedly move on to the exclusive training, only for a boy.

This additional training provides no beneficial results. Rather he is worst off. For starters during his extra training, he creates a mess with urine his mother must clean. His extra training equips him to mess up toilets for the rest of his life. All, because of an unnecessary implementation of the two-step method.

The Two-step Method Messes Up Toilets

The two-step method messes up toilets and yet it remains the hallmark for toilet training boys. It wastes time and is unnecessary. The wiser and smarter choice, is not to receive training, in the first place. That is exactly why unisex toilet training is the only viable solution. It eliminates the extra second-step the, Boot Camp for unsanitary toilets.

What is shocking that despite the irrefutable evidence and long history of unsanitary toilets due to men standing up to urinate. The American Academy of Pediatrics and other leading Child Rearing Practitioners and Experts continues endorsing training boys to stand up to urinate.

Although it is the bedrock for unhygienic and unsanitary and filthy toilets throughout a male's life. In fact, the unsanitary conditions starts furiously during training and becomes a little less during young adulthood. Then returns with regularity in the senior years.

In essence, the mess never stops, but rather goes through different phases and degrees of poor sanitation.

So the defects of standard boys toilet training are numerous and long lasting. It is a defect for the entire life of a male. Unless he changes to unisex toilet retraining and urinating sitting down.

Unisex Toilet Retraining

Open and Shut Case: Urinating Sitting Down

We respectfully submit an open and shut case for unisex toilet retraining and urinating sitting down. This case is easy to prove and decide because the facts are clear.

A review of the evidence shows in many countries unisex toilets and restrooms fulfill an urgent requirement on privacy. There is an increasing aging population and debilitating diseases and deteriorating physical conditions. A common sight today, is a person helping someone of the opposite sex into a Unisex Restroom. Who may be a marriage mate, life-partner, parent, child, caregiver or a friend?

Clearly, gender-specific facilities cannot adequately care for those unique needs and this highlights the urgent need for toilet retraining. Without this process, Unisex Toilets and Restrooms will become filthy like the current Men's Only Restrooms.

The Taiwan environmental protection agency comprehensive research study on 100,000 inspections of public toilets produces conclusive and significant support to that effect.

Key points in favor of urinating sitting down are: urinary frequency. The significant quantities of urine in developed countries and enormous amounts daily worldwide. Also, urination demands one's immediate attention. Any event with such quantities, regularity, and urgency require a sanitary and best practice disposal method.

A fundamental reason for urinating sitting becomes evident with the comparison of a urinal and a home toilet bowl. Urinals, design is specifically for males to stand up and pee in public places. Still, the toilet floor becomes a horrible mess as the Taiwan study supports.

Standing up and urinating at home will also have similar results. This makes sitting down and urinating the practical solution for getting urine directly into the toilet bowl. Without, messing the floor, the toilet seat and the lid and preventing continuous urine cleanups. A, simple unisex method that works for both genders: sitting down and urinating and having clean bathrooms.

The most impressive argument for urinating sitting down is the anatomy of the penis and the urethra. The Men's Health Magazine article by Dr. Levine on why the urethra and the tip of the penis cause urine to go off course.

The second impressive argument is when a male stands up to urinate through his pants fly. The fly pushes up against his urethra and traps his urine. Whereas, when he sits down to urinate and drops his pants his urine flows without restriction.

The picture of the penis under the topic "Milking the Urethra" and the cover of this book provide visuals for further consideration. These confirm why a blind man can sit down and get his urine into the toilet bowl. Better than a person with 20/20 vision standing up to pee in the full light of day.

Another point that argues well for urinating sitting down is this fact. The body eliminates urine in the sitting position when a male sits down to ease his bowels. Therefore, there is only one significant change with retraining. Instead of sitting down only for a bowel movement, he also sits down to urinate.

The various advantages to urinating sitting down include some illnesses and aging. For example, some diseases make men hands and legs tremble, due to weakness and nervousness. So standing up and urinating and holding a penis is difficult. Toilet retraining sitting down and urinating benefits men with those conditions and promotes hygiene and cleanliness.

Taiwan government's proposal for men to sit down to urinate in public toilets: Main objective is to produce better hygiene and cleaner public toilets. This shows concern for men using those toilets. Therefore, in this regard, a man shows less concern for his family when he stands up and pee, at home. Sober reflection on that point is sufficient for accepting the new practice.

The strongest case for urinating sitting down is standard boys' toilet training many defects. These start during potty training and continue throughout a person's life time. Messing the bathroom or toilet starts furiously during toilet training. The mess becomes a little less during young adulthood and adulthood and returns with regularity in the senior years.

Unisex Toilet Retraining

In essence, the mess never stops, but rather goes through different degrees of poor sanitation. The case for urinating standing up rests only on tradition and not any benefits to humans, home or society.

We, the proponents for unisex toilet retraining urinating sitting down; submit evidence that is substantial and undeniable.

This is an open, and a shut case for unisex toilet retraining and urinating sitting down, because doing so produces clean toilets. In contrast, urinating standing up creates smelly filthy unsanitary toilets. A clear case for "changing age-old traditions and meeting 21st Century demands."

Glossary

One-toilet Establishments: These are places with only one toilet or one bathroom and both genders use the same toilet or bathroom or restroom. The main reasons for one-toilet are mostly space limitation and the high cost of gender-specific toilets.

Toilet: Is a sanitation fixture, primarily used by humans in the elimination of their solid body waste, excrement and also their liquid waste, urine. Other names are a bathroom, a toilet, a lavatory or a restroom.

Toilet Different Names: The British calls the room containing the same fixture a toilet or a Loo. In Canada and other areas of North American a bathroom means any room which contain a toilet. In the United States of America, the same facility has the name restroom. In Hong Kong, Australia and Singapore they use the word, toilet.

Unisex: In this definition mean designed for or suitable to both sexes and not distinguished between male and female. So both genders are able to use it.

Unisex Public Toilet: This is a gender neutral toilet and it also goes by the name unisex toilet, family toilet, unisex bathroom, unisex restroom and gender neutral bathroom.

Unisex Toilet: This is a toilet or bathroom or restroom or lavatory used by both genders. Therefore, by definition, the home toilet is a unisex toilet and also toilets on buses, trains, airplanes, bars, some hotels, restaurants, small businesses and small offices.

Unisex Toilet Retraining: This is a new concept the author pioneered. It means the process males retrain to use the toilet changing from the standard urinating standing up to urinating sitting down. Plus, the learning of new skills that promote good hygiene and clean toilets and bathrooms.

Urinal: Is a special toilet males use for urinating. It has the form of a container or simply a wall, with drainage and automatic or manual flushing.

About the Author

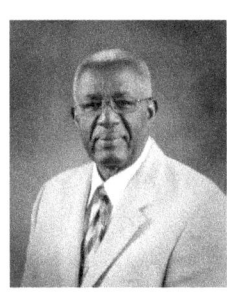

At the age of 25 years, the author arrives in New York City, USA. He visits private residences and smells human urine odors in toilets. He hates the scent.

One day to his surprise he stands up to pee and sees his urine missing the toilet bowl and falling on the floor. On subsequent occasions, as his first squirt misses the toilet bowl he tries various techniques. Stop urinating and start again, thinking his urine stream will self-correct. Another strategy stop urinating and start pinching the tip of his penis and begin urinating again. Reasoning his urine flow would become laser-like and go straight into the bowl. These were unsuccessful, and did not prevent his urine from going on the bathroom floor.

One day, in 1968, his urine fell on his feet. That was the limit. He said, enough and retrained himself in urinating sitting down.

Unisex Toilet Retraining

In February, 2013, he sees articles on the proposals for legislation in Sweden and Taiwan: countries encouraging men to sit down in public toilets to urinate and have clean toilets.

This interests him; because it is the exact reason why he urinates sitting down. He researches the topic and discovers the main reasons why a male's urine goes off track. Are because, of the tip of the penis, and the urethra. This new understanding impresses him because of this fundamental point. When a male stands up and urinates there is the high probability of squirting urine in the toilet.

He reflects on these truths. Women urinate sitting down and have clean toilets. His retraining and sitting down produces the same results. Thus, he concludes millions of men worldwide who stand up and urinate needs retraining in the same clean method, urinating sitting down.

Since the method works for male and female he pioneers Unisex Toilet Retraining and writes this book. Unisex Toilet Retraining Urinating Sitting Down Produces Clean Toilets. Urinating Standing Up Creates Smelly Filthy Unsanitary Toilets.

The author knows toilet retraining works. Because, four and a half decades after his personal retraining, he still sits down to urinate and have a clean toilet at home. This pleases his wife because just like him, she also hates smelly human urine odors in toilets.

Anthony Seymour Browne was born in Barbados and he lived in Montserrat and the U.S.A. Graduate of Bernard M. Baruch College, the City University of New York, with a BBA Degree in Accounting. An Ordained Minister as of June 12, 1993 and he follows Jesus Christ's model. After 32 years in America Anthony returns to

Barbados where he presently resides with his wife, the former Wendy Franklin.

Unisex Toilet Retraining